Paramedics

by Julie Murray

Dash!
LEVELED READERS
An Imprint of Abdo Zoom • abdobooks.com

2

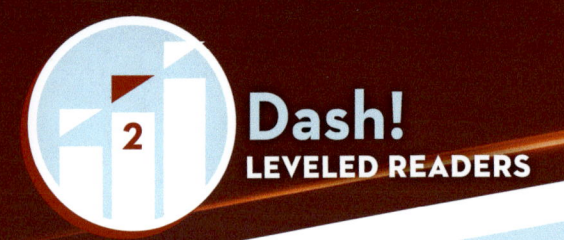

Dash!
LEVELED READERS

Level 1 – Beginning
Short and simple sentences with familiar words or patterns for children who are beginning to understand how letters and sounds go together.

Level 2 – Emerging
Longer words and sentences with more complex language patterns for readers who are practicing common words and letter sounds.

Level 3 – Transitional
More developed language and vocabulary for readers who are becoming more independent.

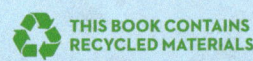
THIS BOOK CONTAINS RECYCLED MATERIALS

abdobooks.com

Published by Abdo Zoom, a division of ABDO, PO Box 398166, Minneapolis, Minnesota 55439. Copyright © 2021 by Abdo Consulting Group, Inc. International copyrights reserved in all countries. No part of this book may be reproduced in any form without written permission from the publisher. Dash!™ is a trademark and logo of Abdo Zoom.

Printed in China.
102020
012021

Photo Credits: Alamy, Getty Images, iStock, Shutterstock
Production Contributors: Kenny Abdo, Jennie Forsberg, Grace Hansen, John Hansen
Design Contributors: Dorothy Toth, Neil Klinepier, Laura Graphenteen

Library of Congress Control Number: 2020910903

Publisher's Cataloging in Publication Data

Names: Murray, Julie, author.
Title: Paramedics / by Julie Murray
Description: Minneapolis, Minnesota : Abdo Zoom, 2021 | Series: Emergency jobs | Includes online resources and index.
Identifiers: ISBN 9781098223083 (lib. bdg.) | ISBN 9781098223786 (ebook) | ISBN 9781098224134 (Read-to-Me ebook)
Subjects: LCSH: Emergency medical technicians--Juvenile literature. | EMTs (Medicine)--Juvenile literature. | First responders--Juvenile literature. | Assistance in emergencies--Juvenile literature.
Classification: DDC 363.3481--dc23

Table of Contents

Paramedics

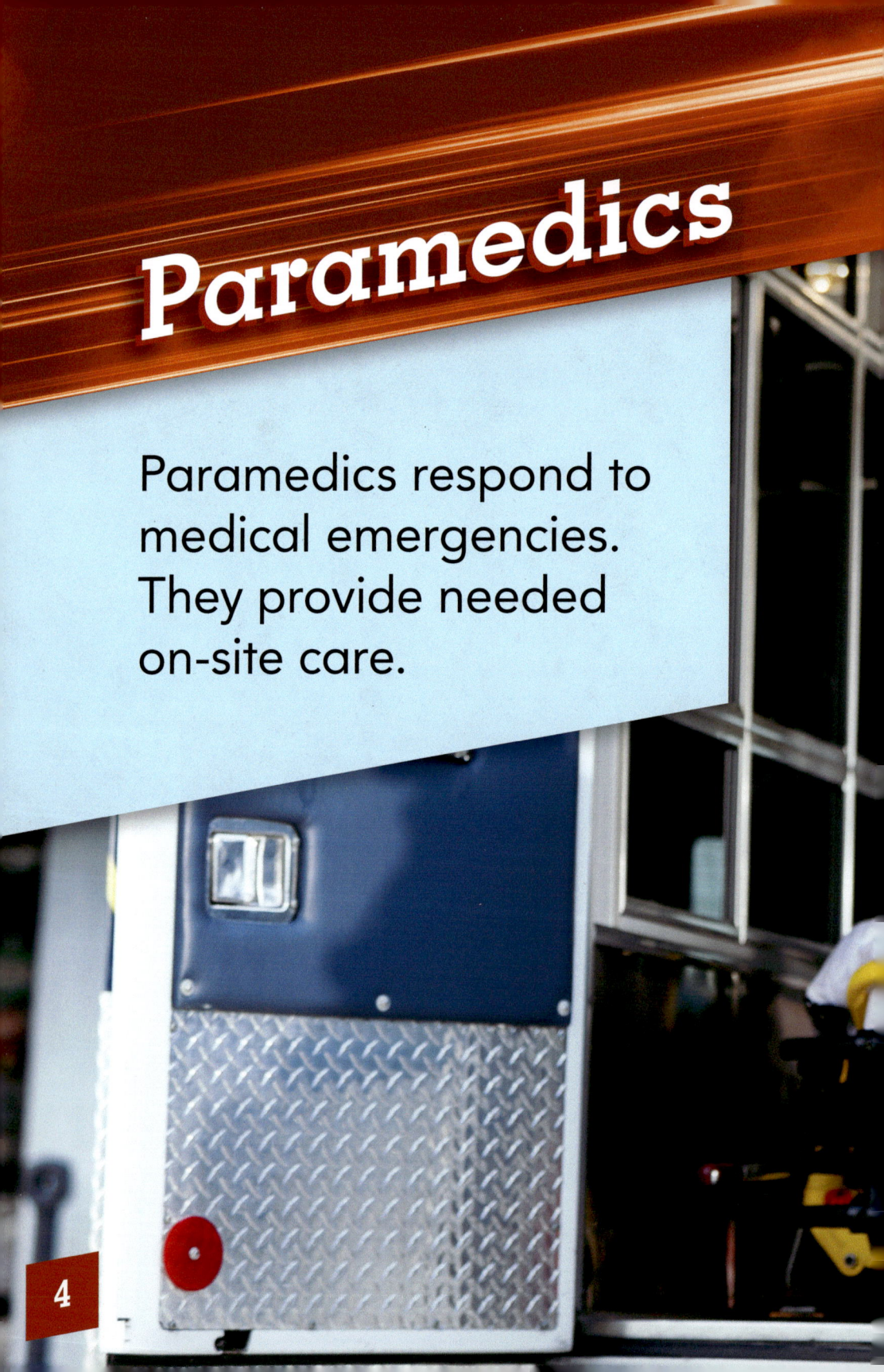

Paramedics respond to medical emergencies. They provide needed on-site care.

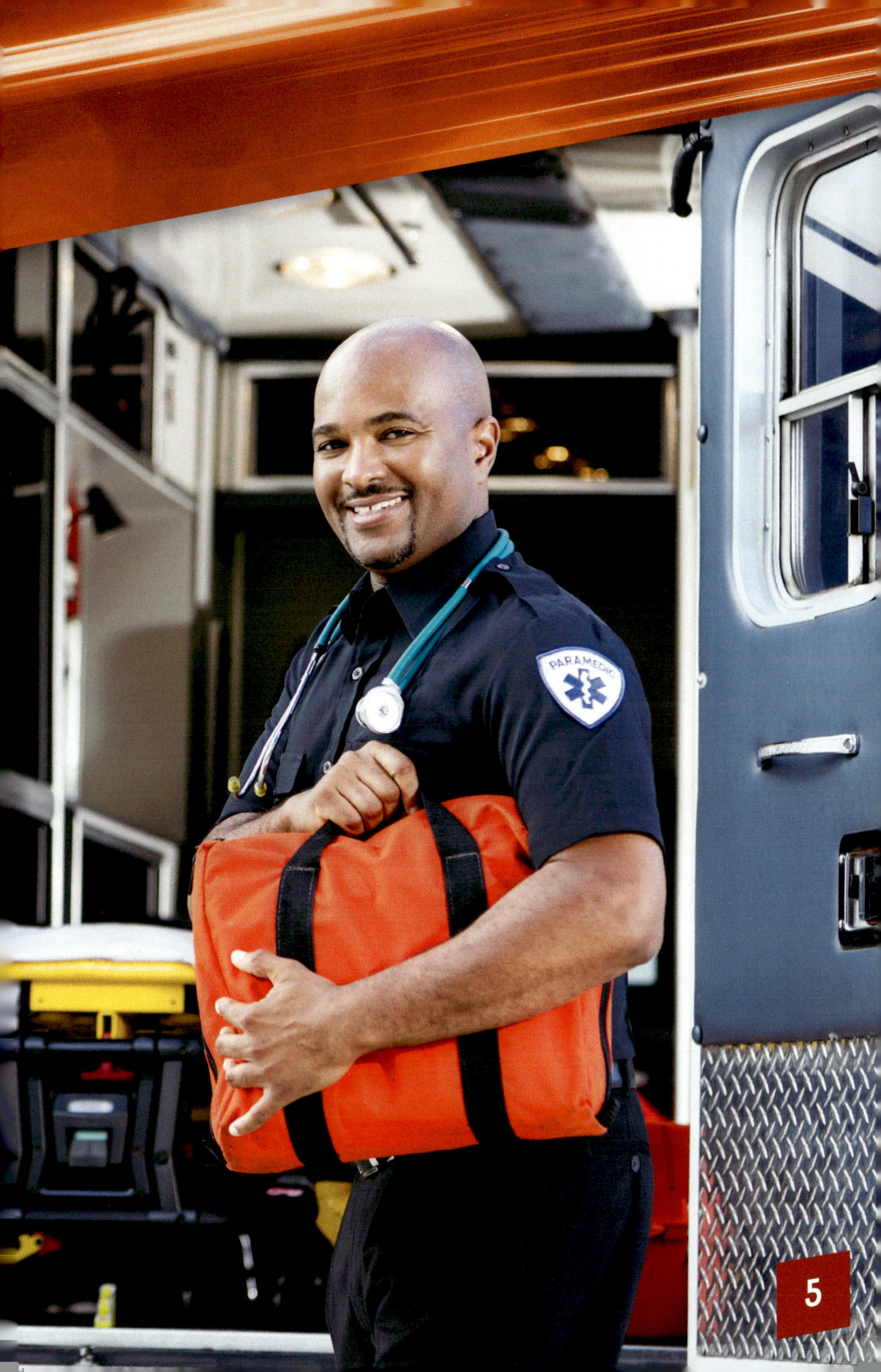

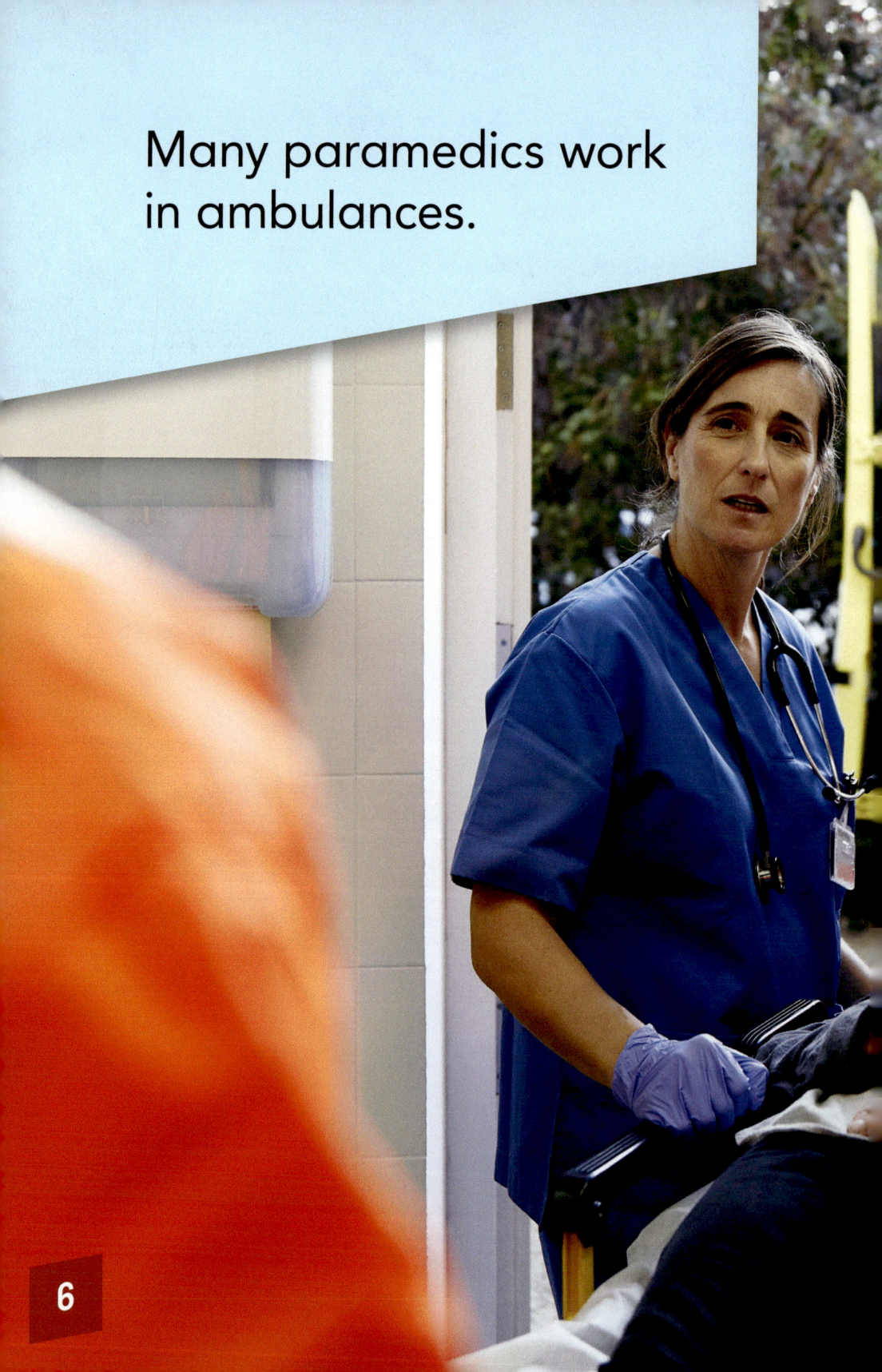

Many paramedics work in ambulances.

6

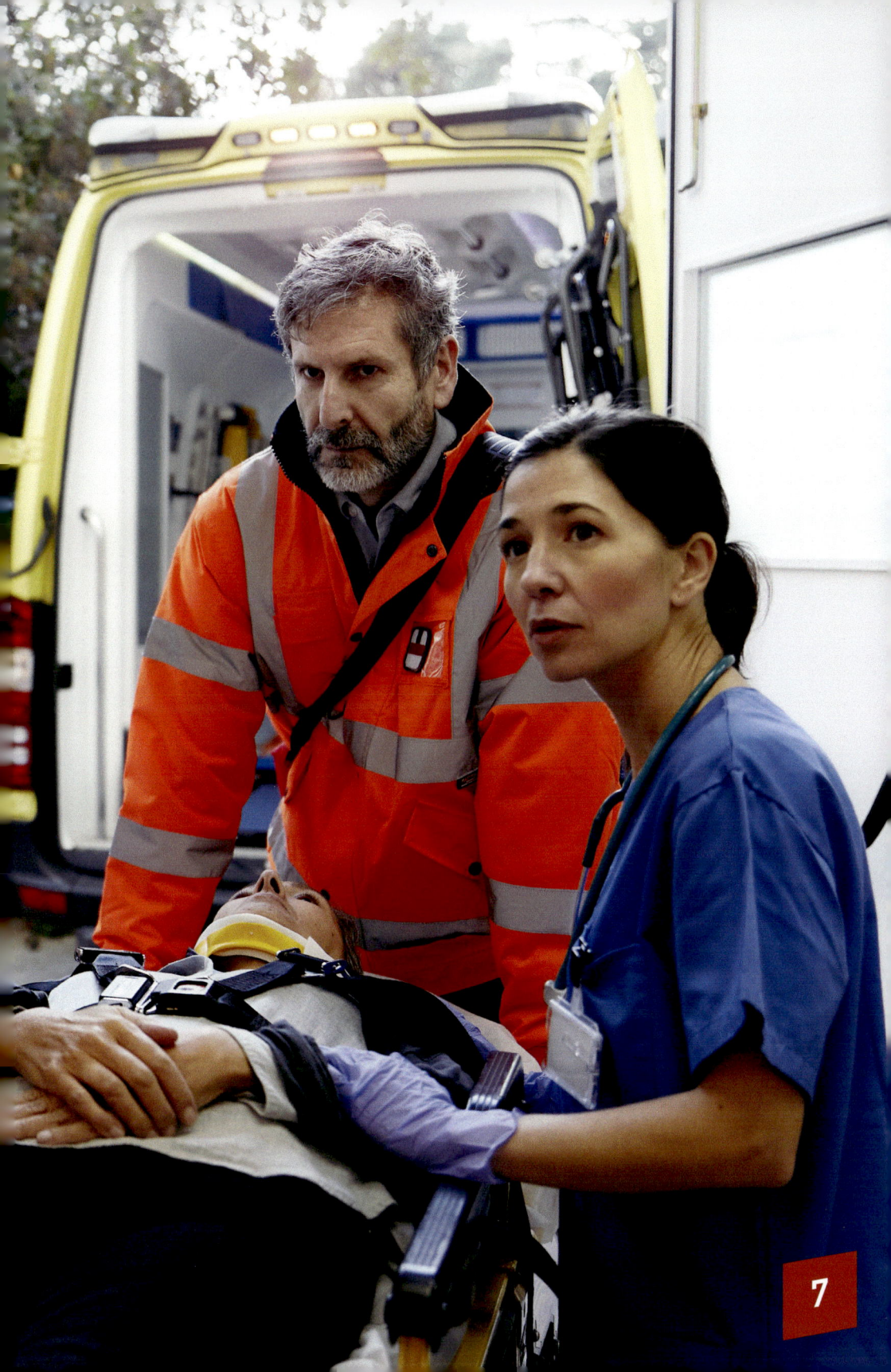

7

They help at car accident scenes. They treat the injured.

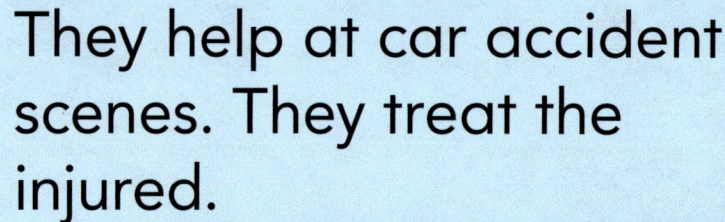

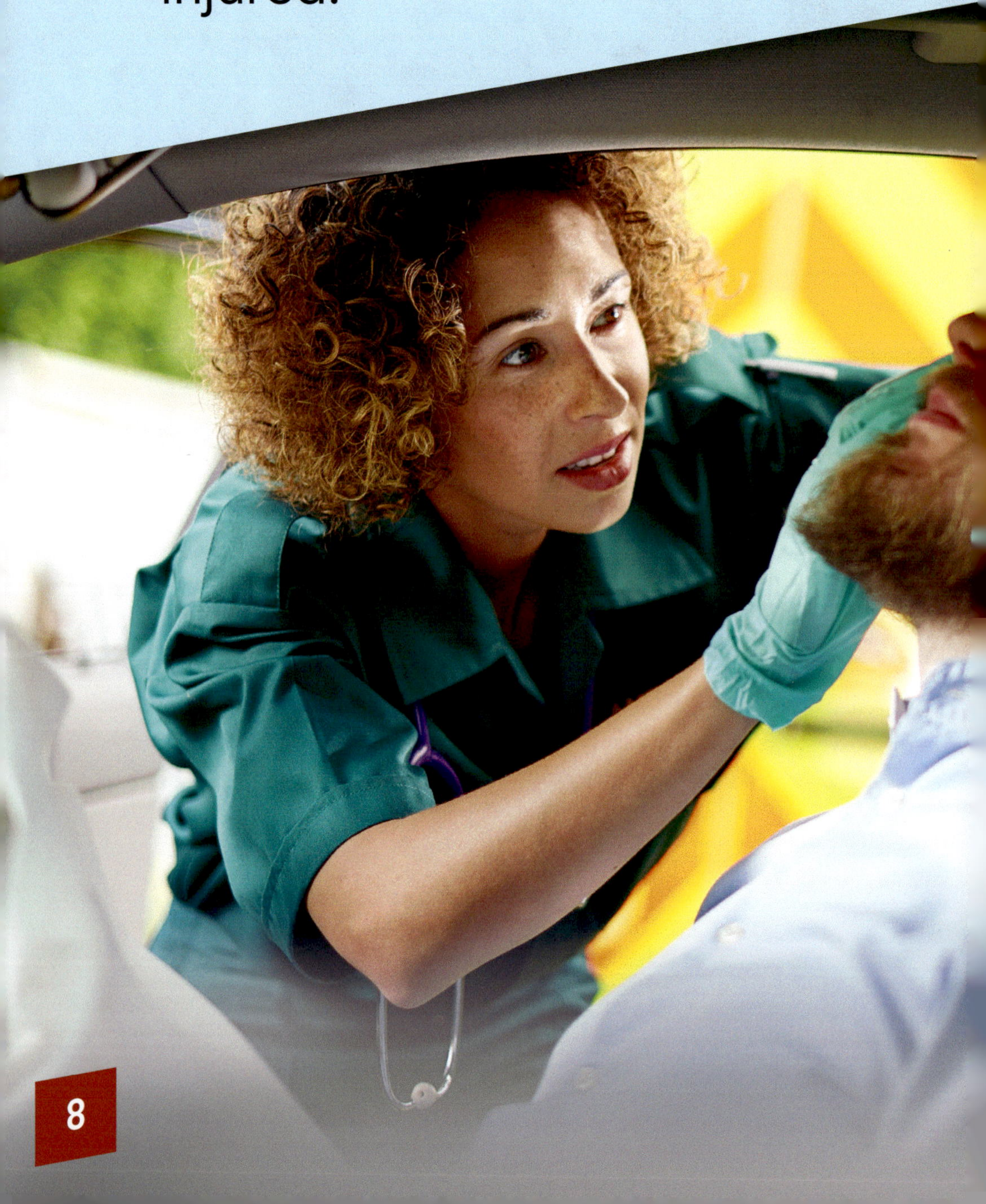

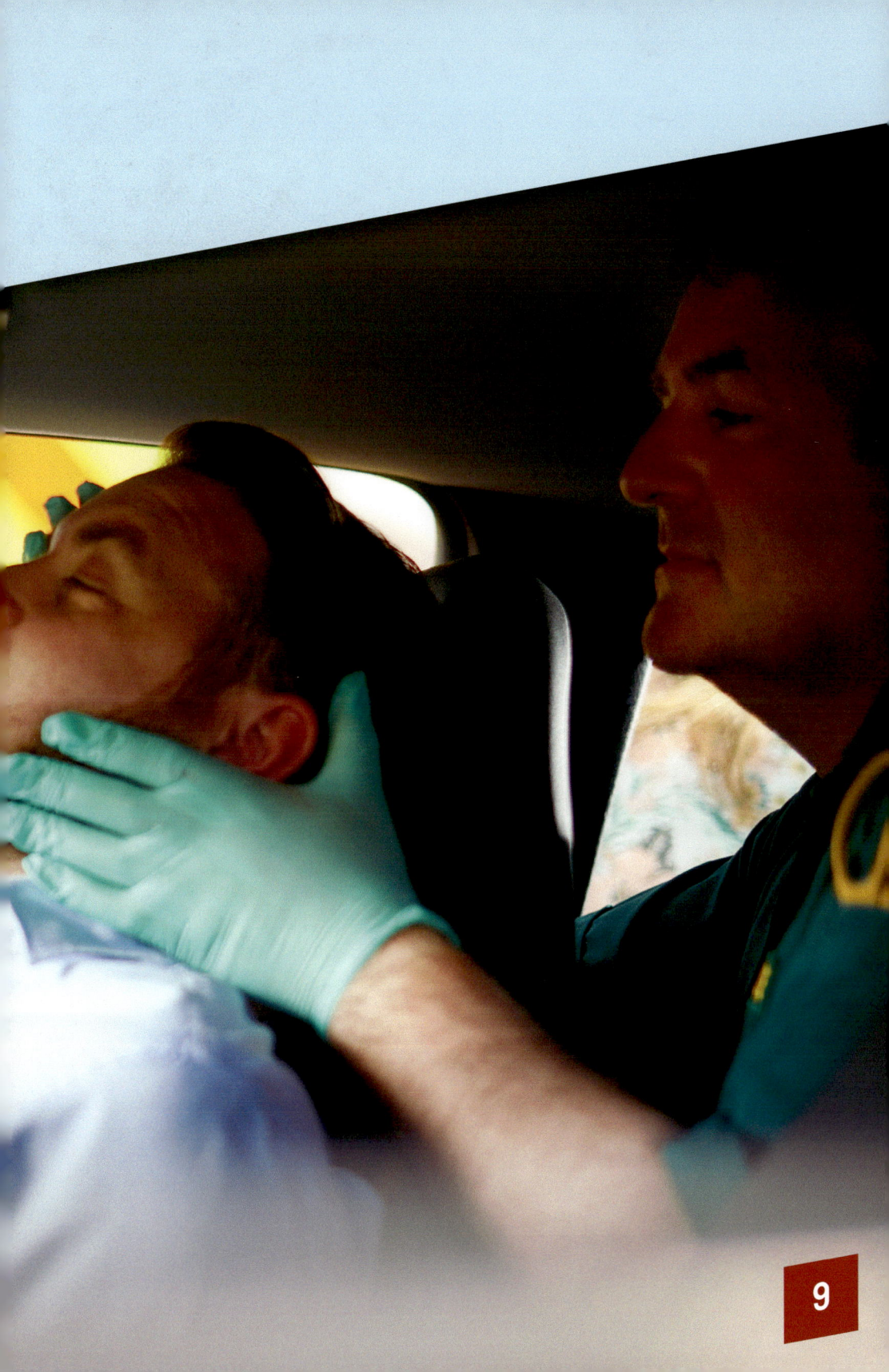

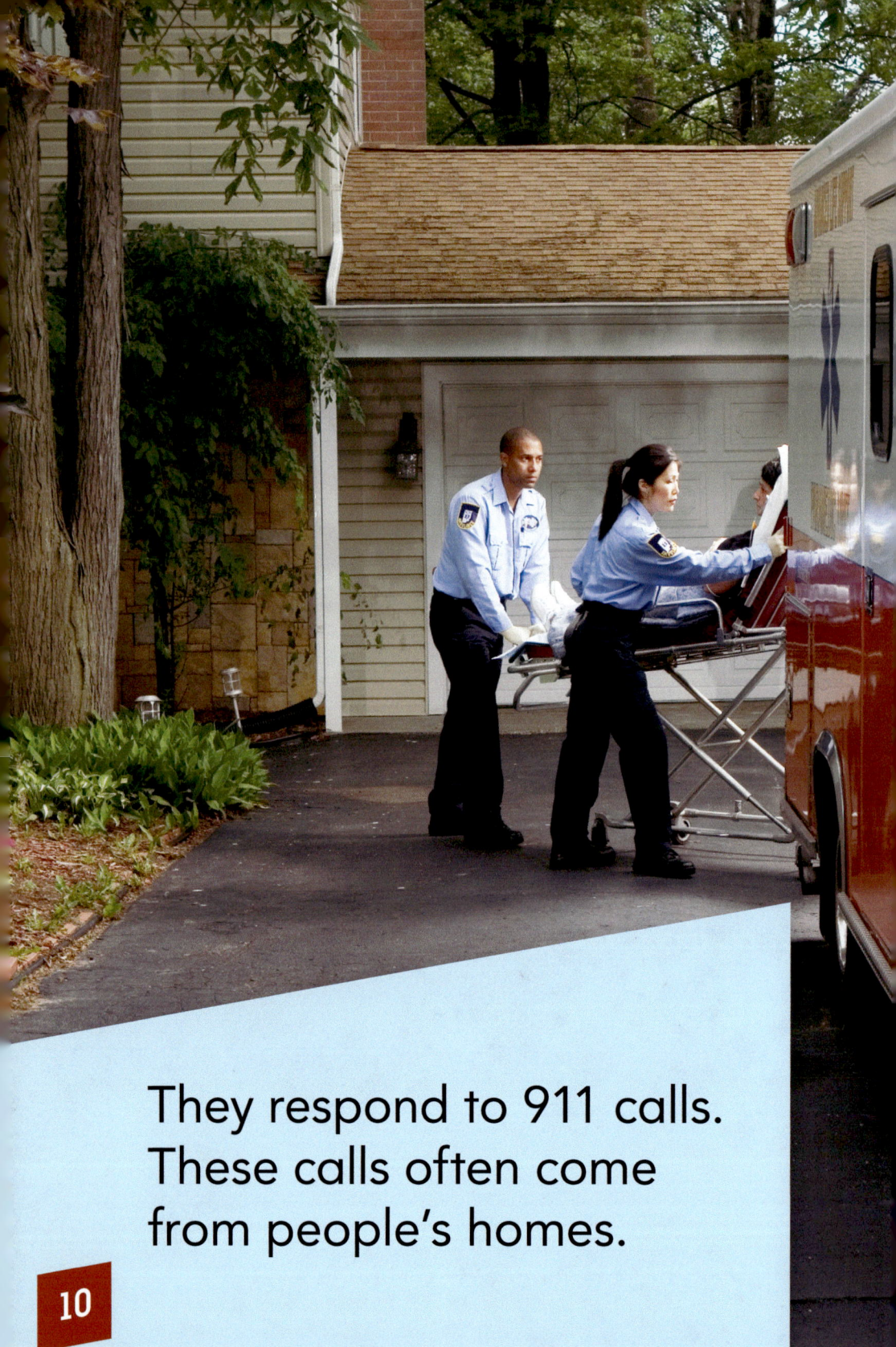

They respond to 911 calls.
These calls often come
from people's homes.

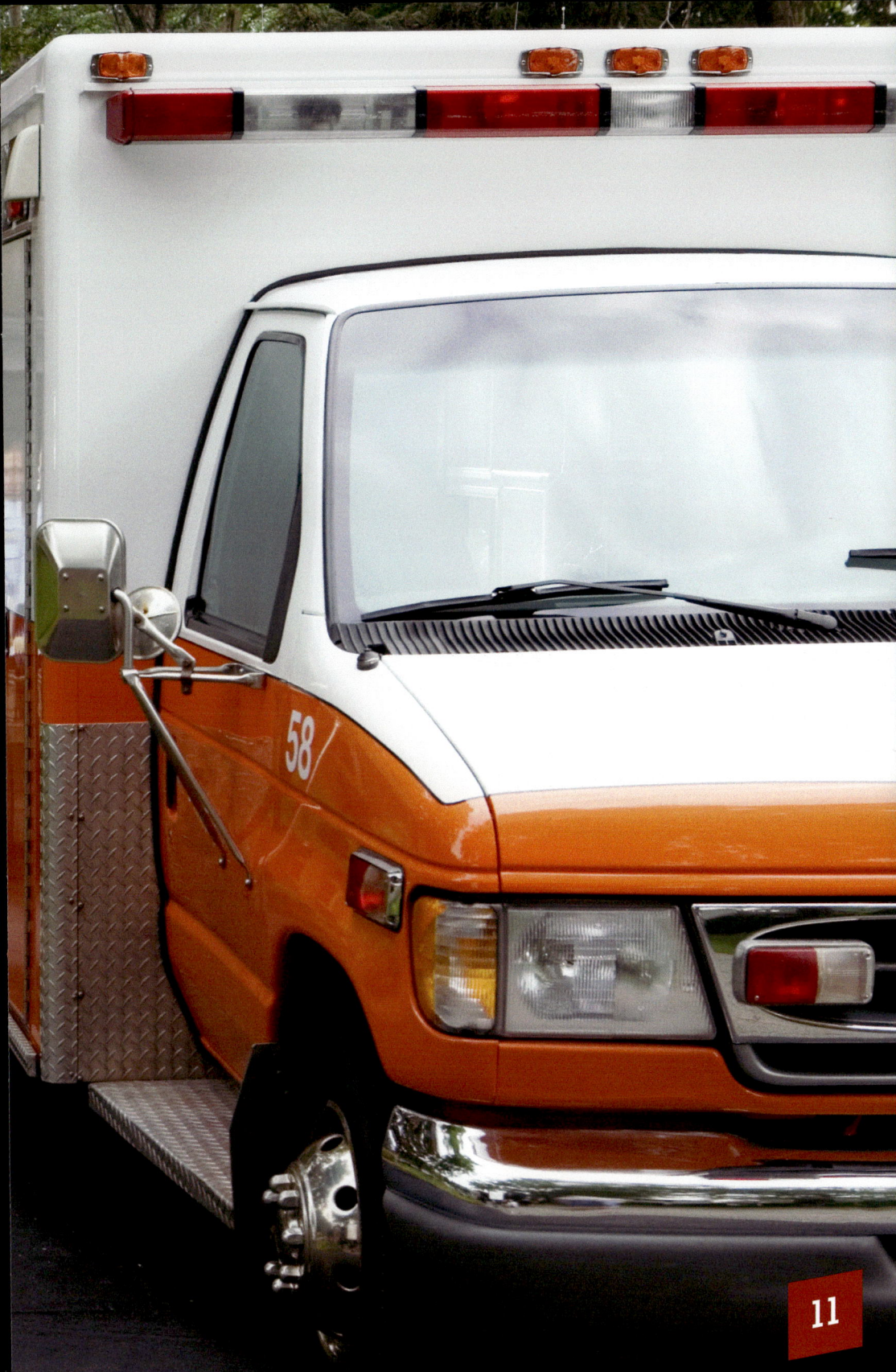

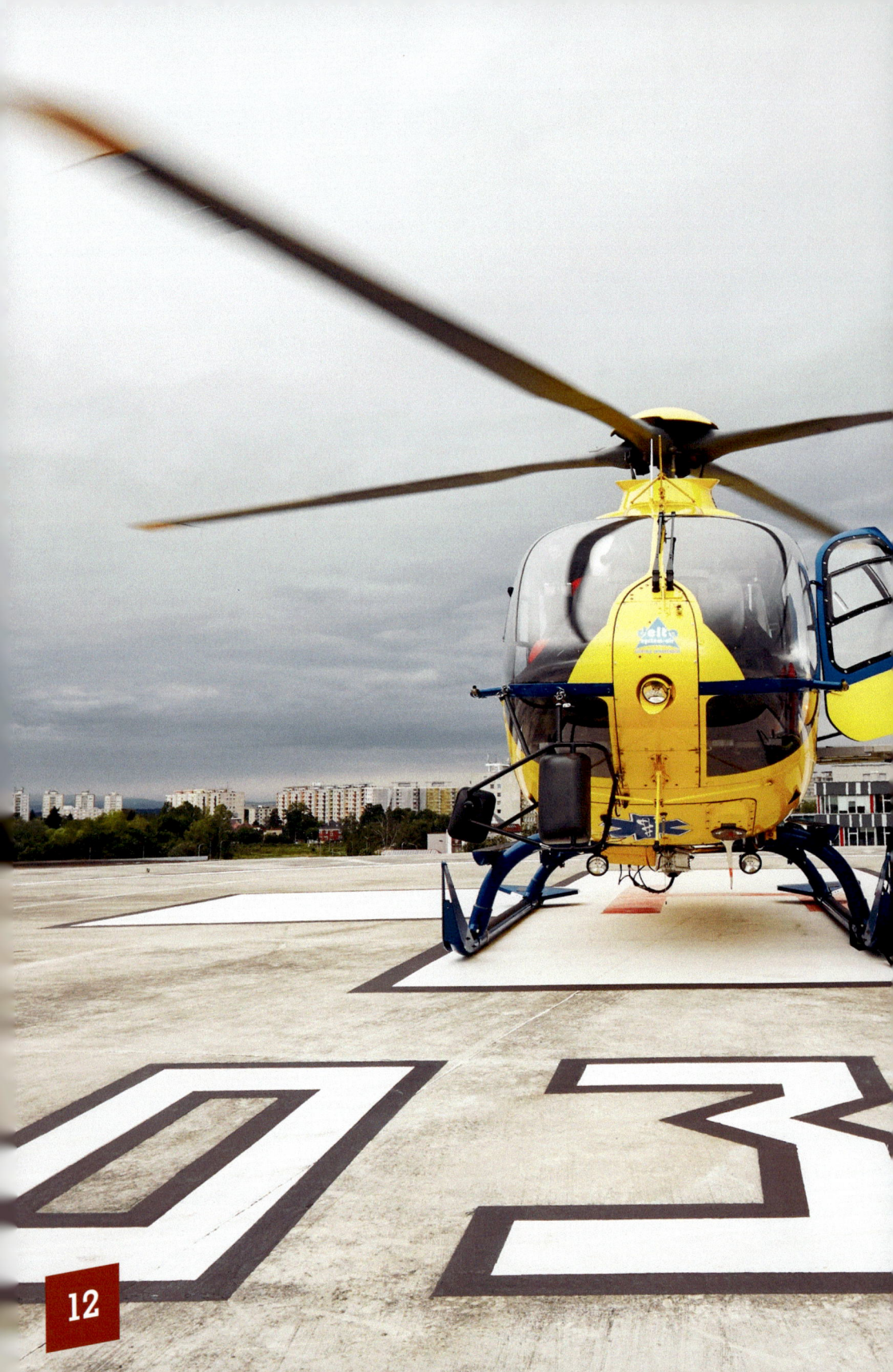

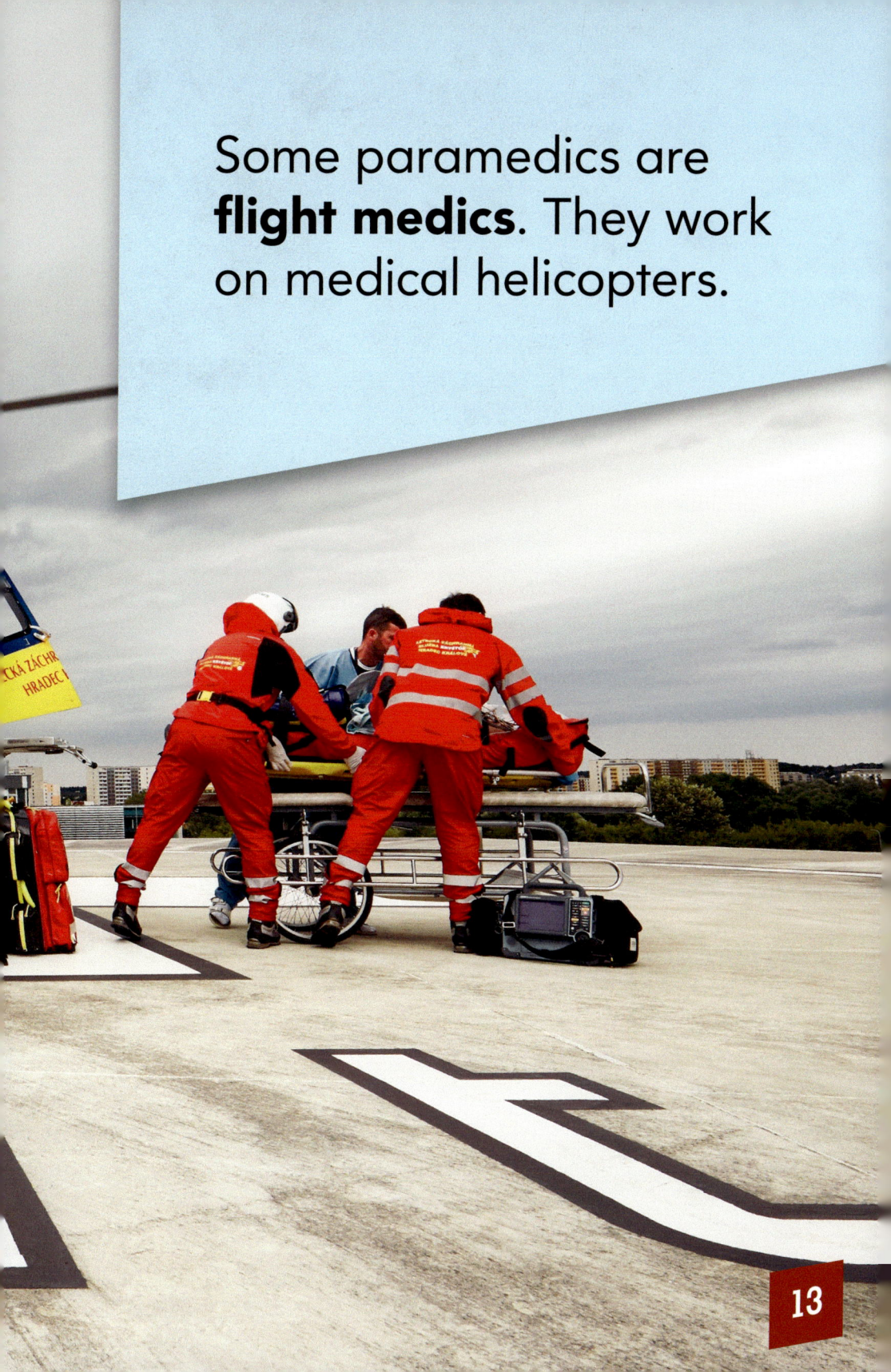

Some paramedics are **flight medics**. They work on medical helicopters.

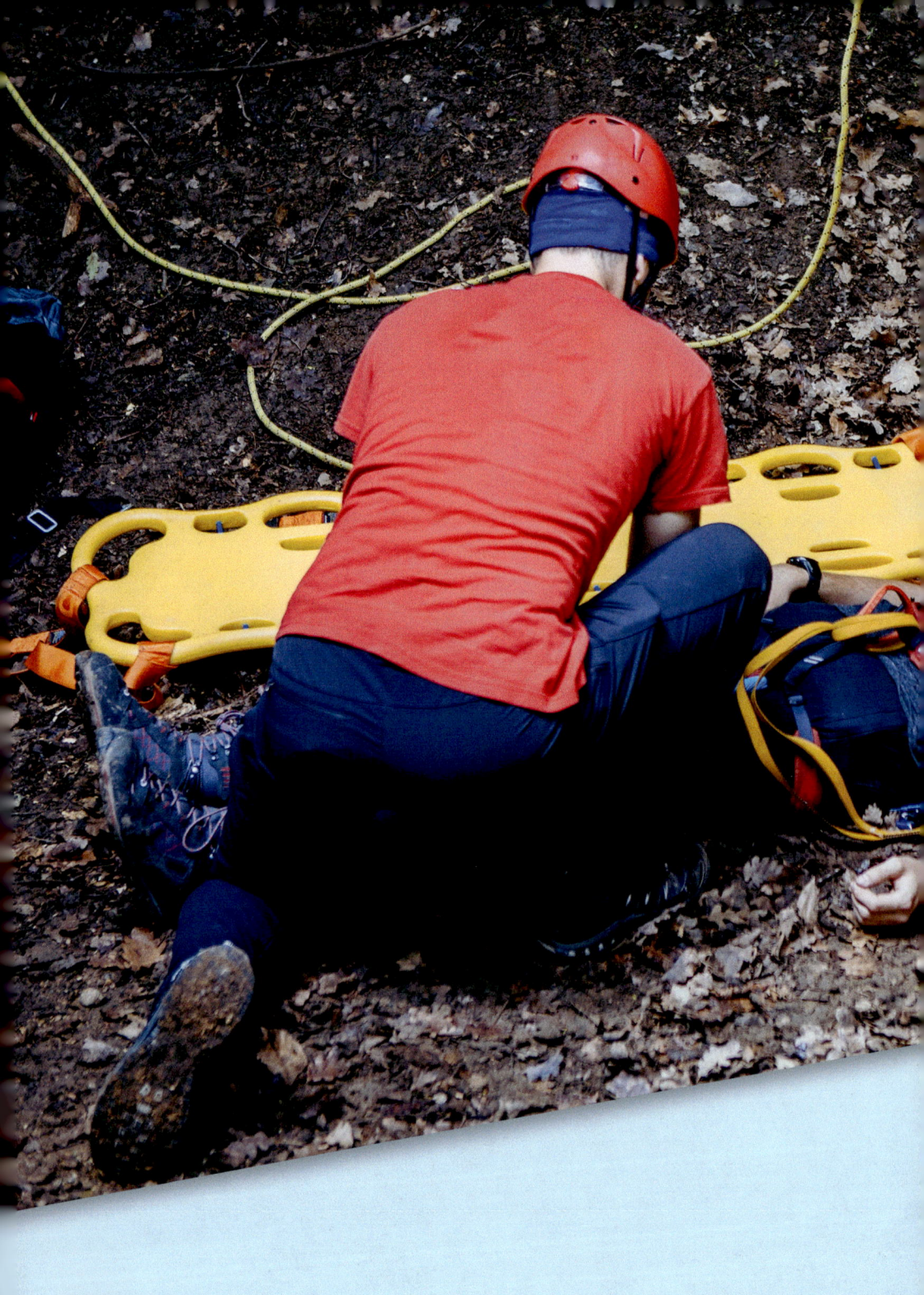

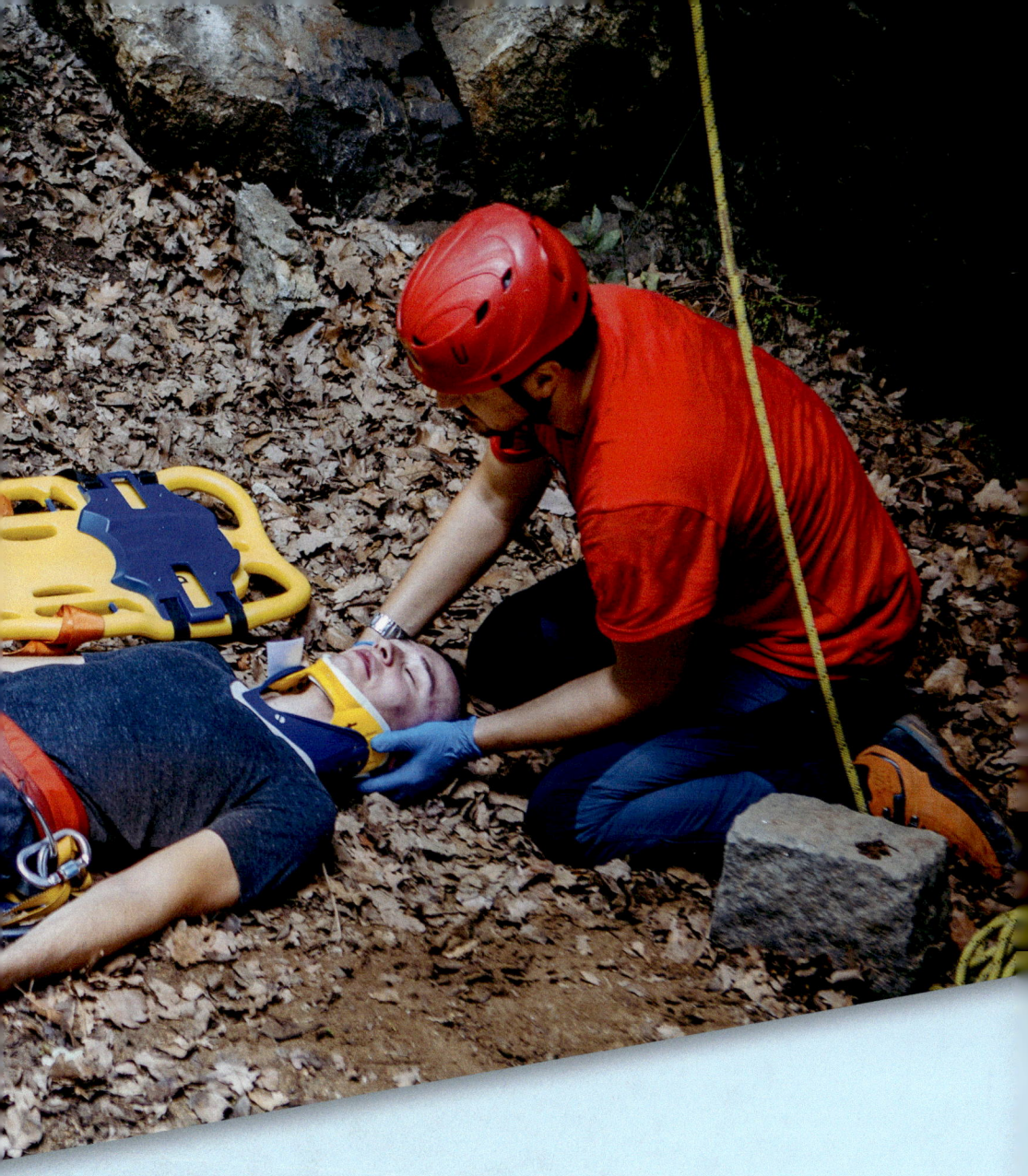

Others work with search-and-rescue teams. They check to make sure the rescued people are OK.

Training

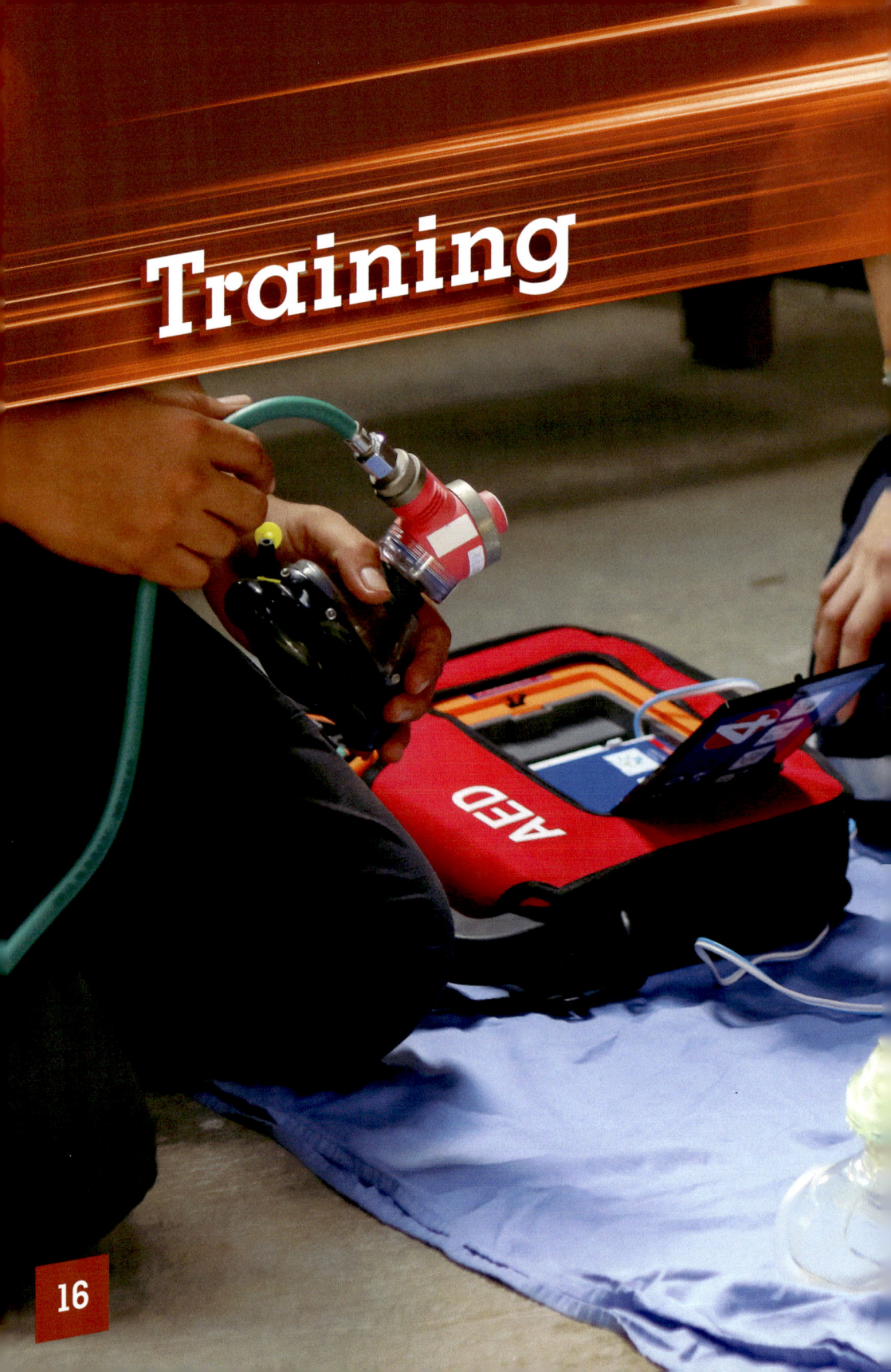

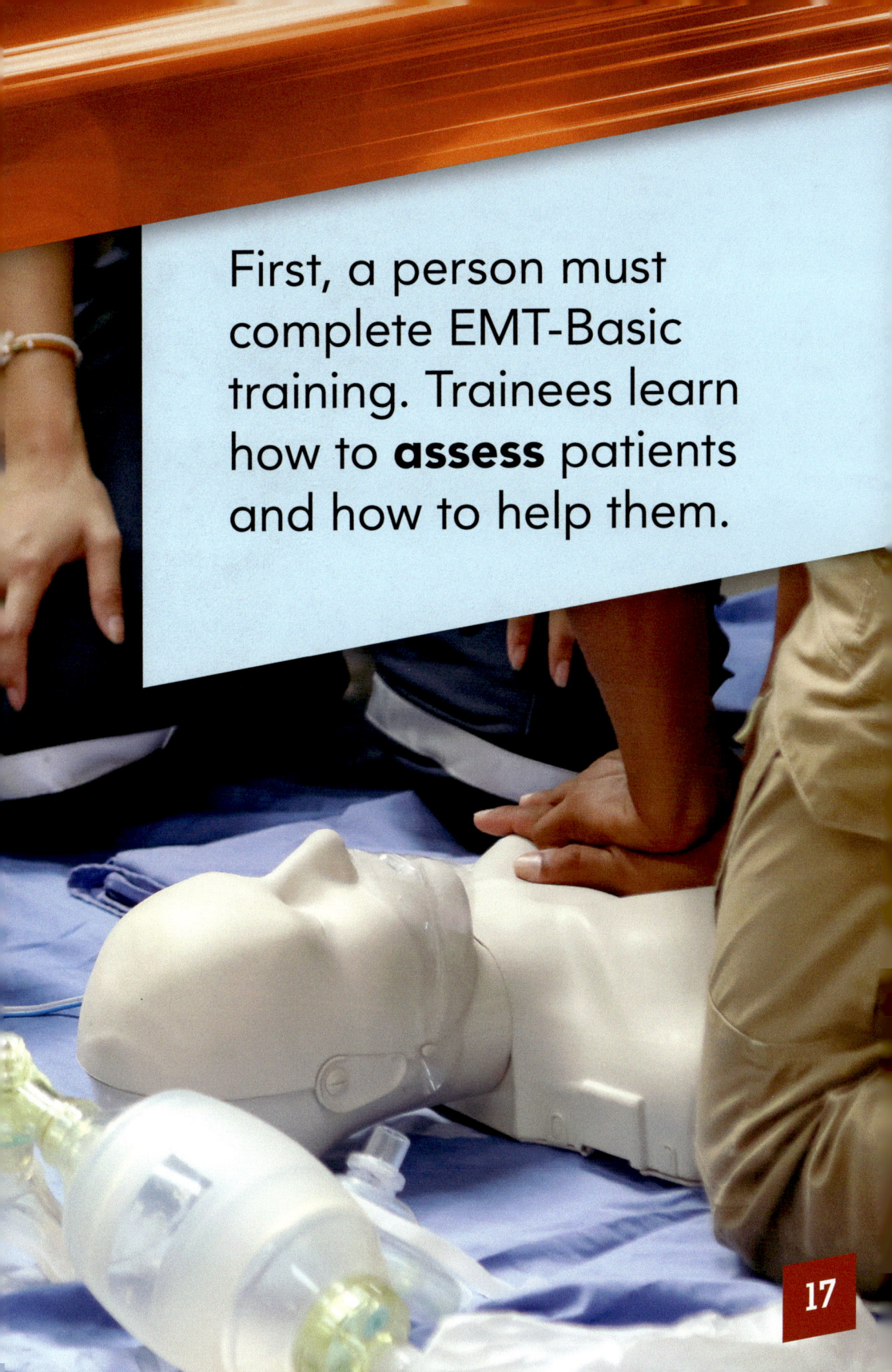

First, a person must complete EMT-Basic training. Trainees learn how to **assess** patients and how to help them.

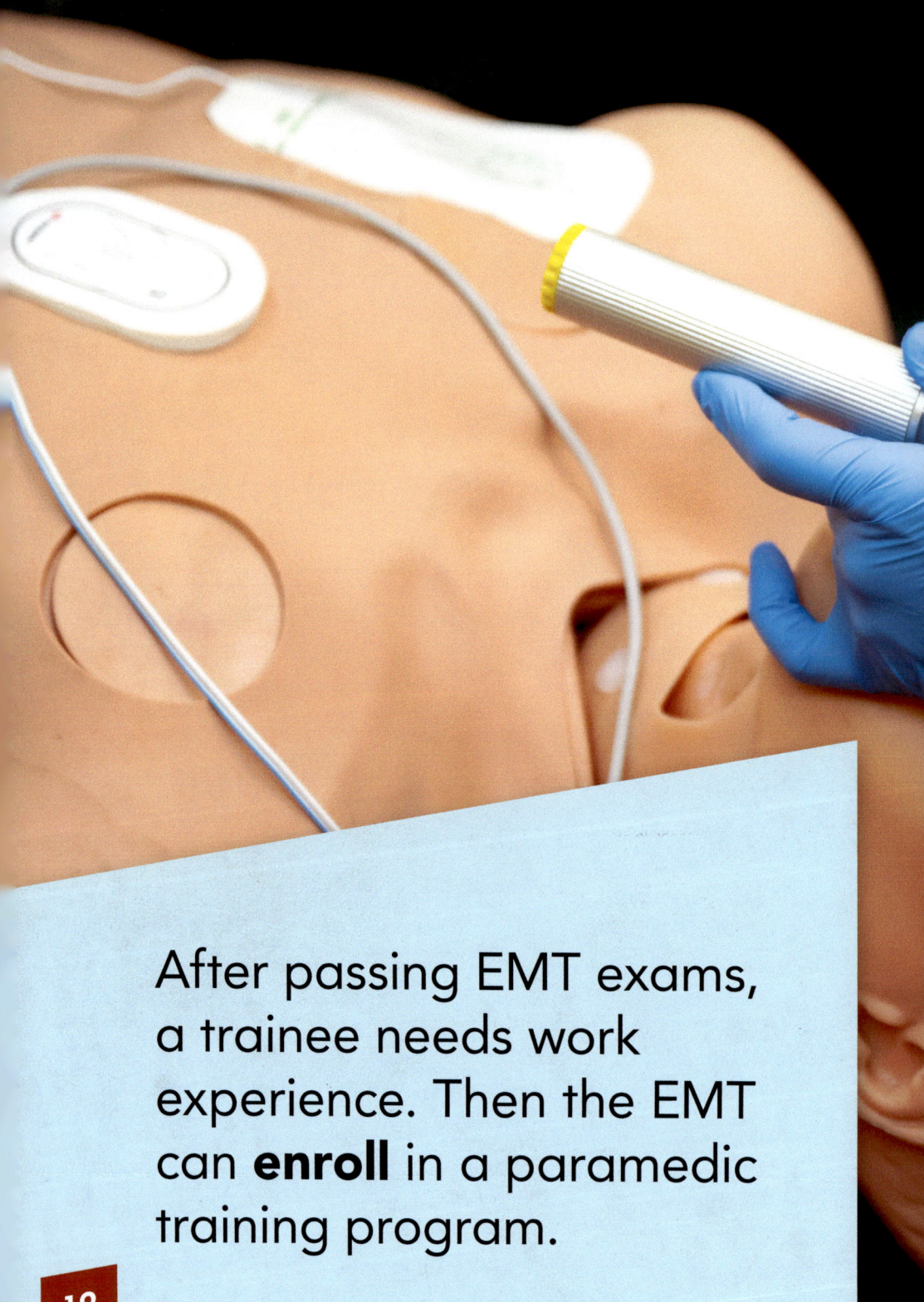

After passing EMT exams, a trainee needs work experience. Then the EMT can **enroll** in a paramedic training program.

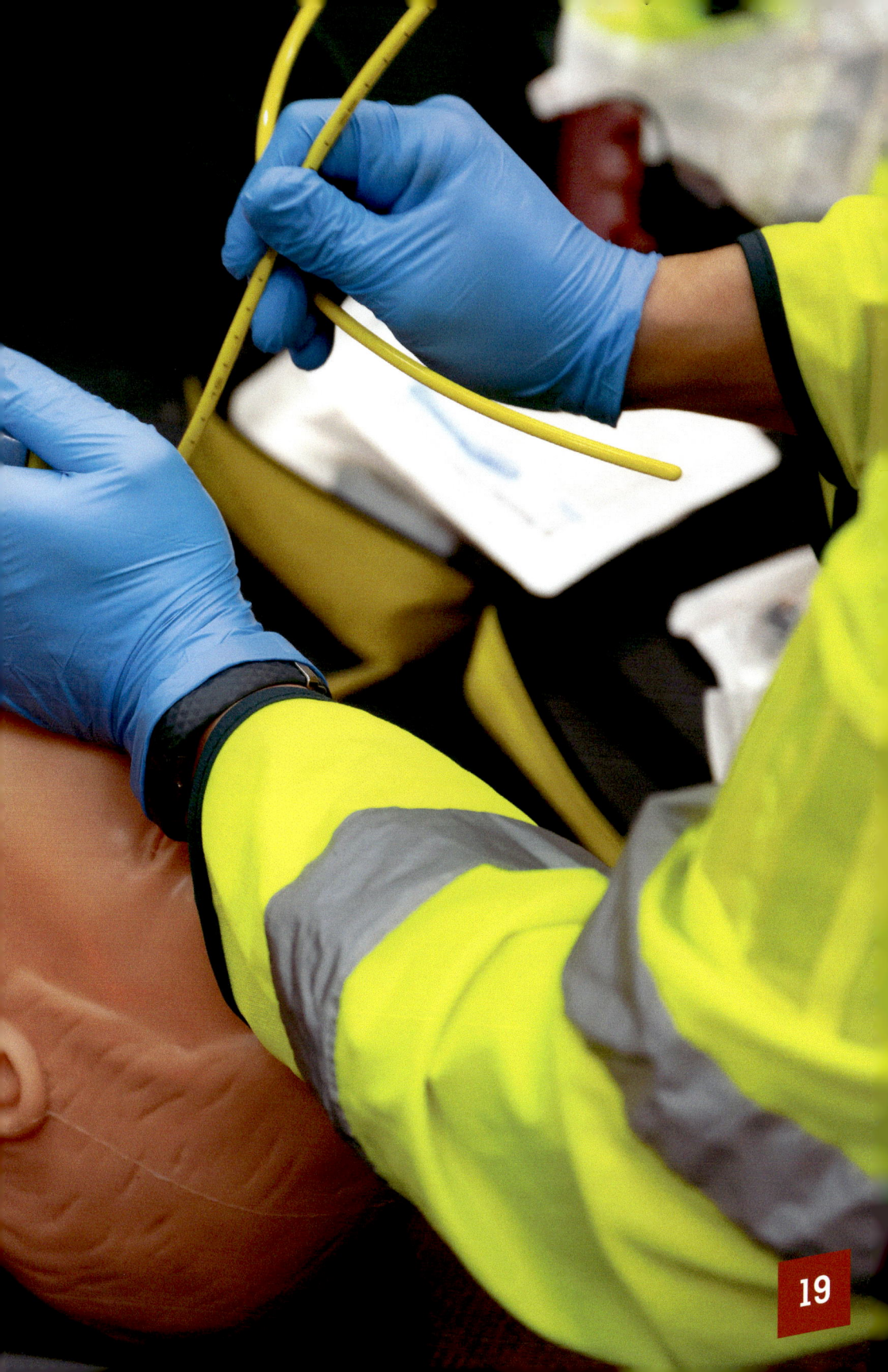

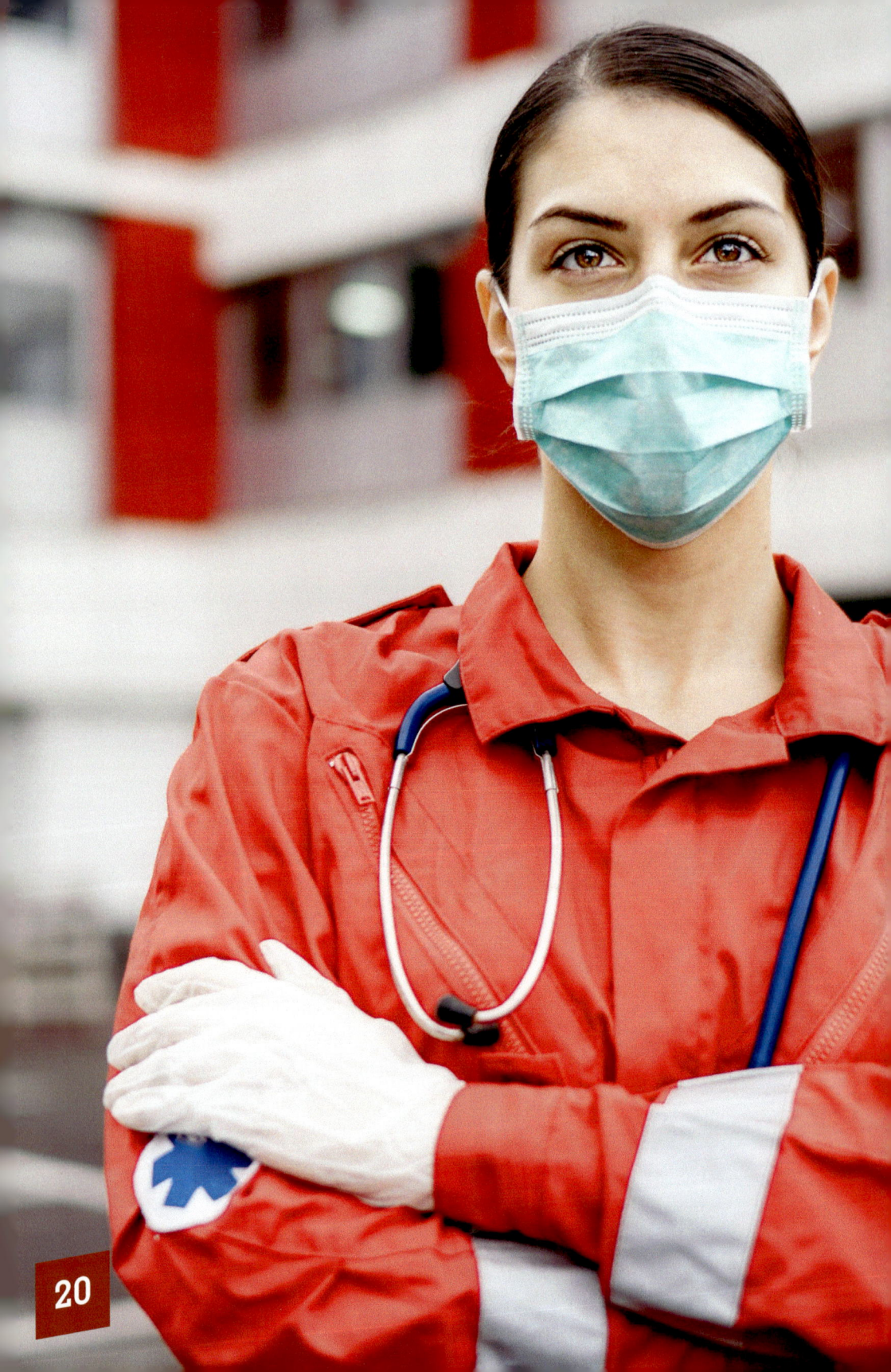

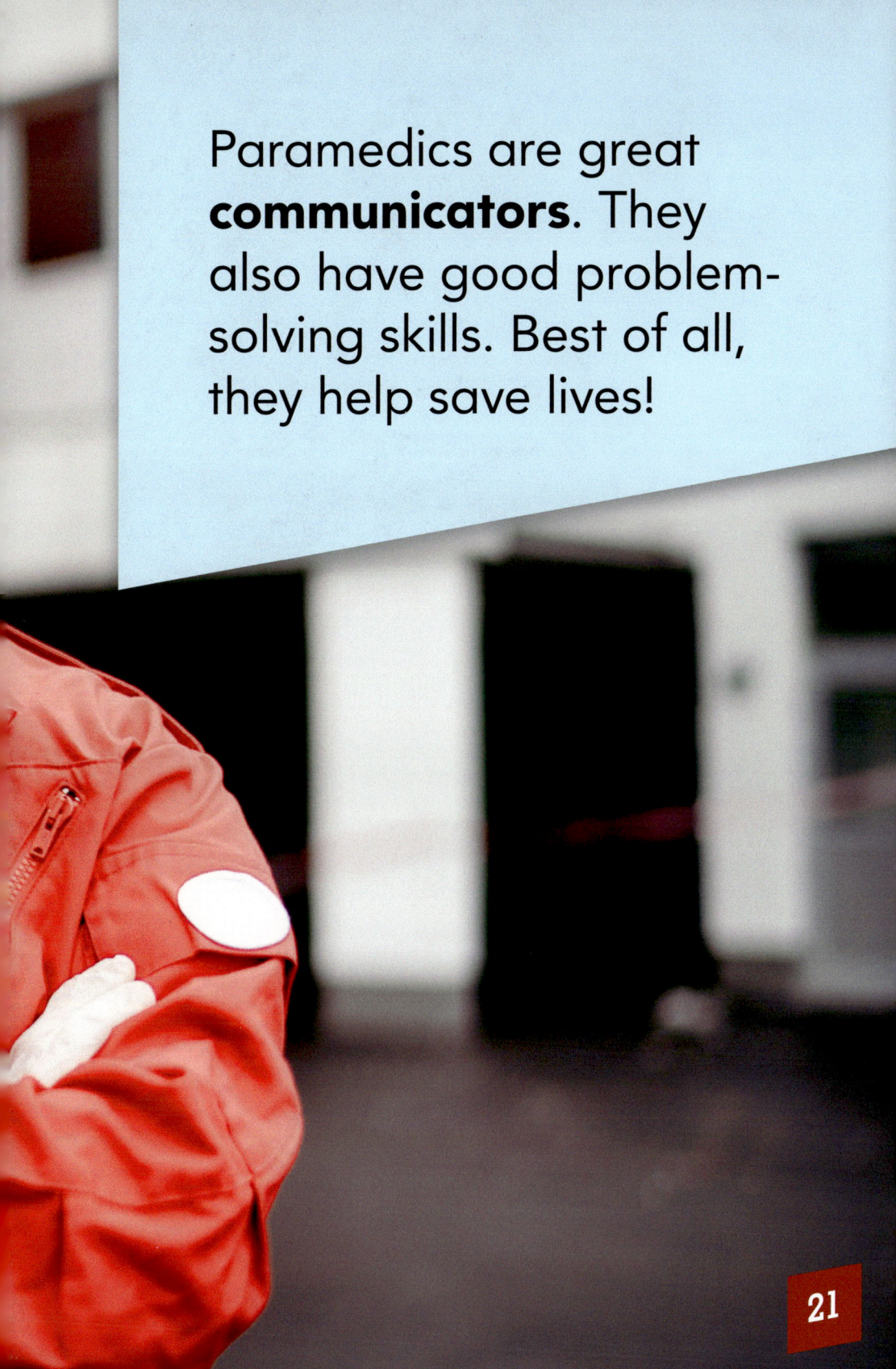

Paramedics are great **communicators**. They also have good problem-solving skills. Best of all, they help save lives!

More Facts

- There are more than 260,000 EMTs and paramedics in the United States.

- Many paramedics work for their city's fire department.

- The Miami Fire Department had the first paramedic program. It was started in 1969.

Glossary

assess – to look at and try to learn the seriousness of something, like an injury.

communicator – one who expresses thoughts, ideas, or information.

enroll – sign up officially.

flight medic – or flight paramedic, a highly trained paramedic that provides care to sick and injured patients while they are transferred via aircraft.

Index

accidents 8

ambulance 6

duties 4, 8, 10, 13, 15, 21

education 17, 18

flight medics 13

helicopter 13

injuries 8

search and rescue 15

Online Resources

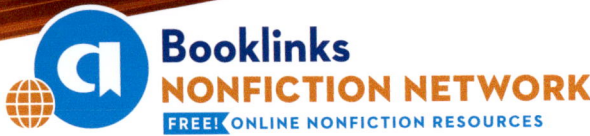

Booklinks
NONFICTION NETWORK
FREE! ONLINE NONFICTION RESOURCES

To learn more about paramedics, please visit **abdobooklinks.com** or scan this QR code. These links are routinely monitored and updated to provide the most current information available.